My Body Is Mine,
My Feelings Are Mine

A Storybook About Body Safety for Young Children
with an Adult Guidebook

By Susan Hoke, LCSW, ACSW
Illustrated by Bruce Van Patter

Note to the adult: We recommend reading the adult guidelines beginning on page 55 before you read this storybook with young children. When reading this storybook, encourage children to respond to the characters and discuss their thoughts and feelings.

Published by:
Childswork/Childsplay, LLC
Plainview, N.Y.

My Body is Mine, My Feelings are Mine

By Susan Hoke, LCSW, ACSW
Illustrated by Bruce Van Patter
Designed by Charles Brenna

Published by:

Childswork/Childsplay, LLC
A Division of The Bureau
Plainview, N.Y. For At-Risk Youth
Phone: 1-800-962-1141

Childswork/Childsplay is a catalog and publisher of products for mental health professionals, teachers, and parents who wish to help children with their social and emotional growth.

ISBN 1-882732-24-3

Fourth Printing

With love for:
Katie, Frankie, Ginny, Amanda, Sam and Danielle

Foreword

The number of children who are affected by sexual abuse continues to astound and confound our society. As parents, teachers, and mental health professionals, it is our first and primary job to keep children safe; but too often, we fail in this most basic of tasks.

For better or worse, even young children in today's society must learn to keep themselves safe from harm. They must learn what are appropriate kinds of "touching" and what are not. They must learn the danger signs that indicate when someone is trying to exploit their innocence, and they must learn what to do if that happens.

Susan Hoke has written a wonderfully engaging book for young children to teach them the most important information about protecting themselves from the possibility of sexual abuse. In addition, she has written a thoughtful guideline for adults, which summarizes the major points that parents and professionals should know in order to prevent sexual abuse from occurring, and responding appropriately if it does.

Readers should be aware, however, that this book is just a jumping-off point for dealing with this difficult topic. The storybook will introduce the basic concept of body safety to children, but it is only a source of information, not some magical suit of armor. Parents and teachers must make time to keep the dialogue open about this important topic, and to always make children feel that they can speak openly and honestly about their concerns.

Similarly, the adult section is only designed to present the basic guidelines of identifying the occurrence of sexual abuse and responding in ways which are most likely to protect the child from further harm. Teachers of young children, in particular, must appreciate the complexity of helping children where abuse has been suspected, and should immediately consult qualified and impartial professionals to guide them through the maze of legal, ethical, and psychological issues.

-Lawrence E. Shapiro, Ph.D.

CONTENTS

"Hey! Hey you! I bet you can't finnnnnnnnnd me! When you turn that page I bet you can't finnnnnnnd me!"

That must be Lilli talking. She loves to play hide and seek. Lilli just learned something important about safety. She might even tell us if we find her! You look over there.

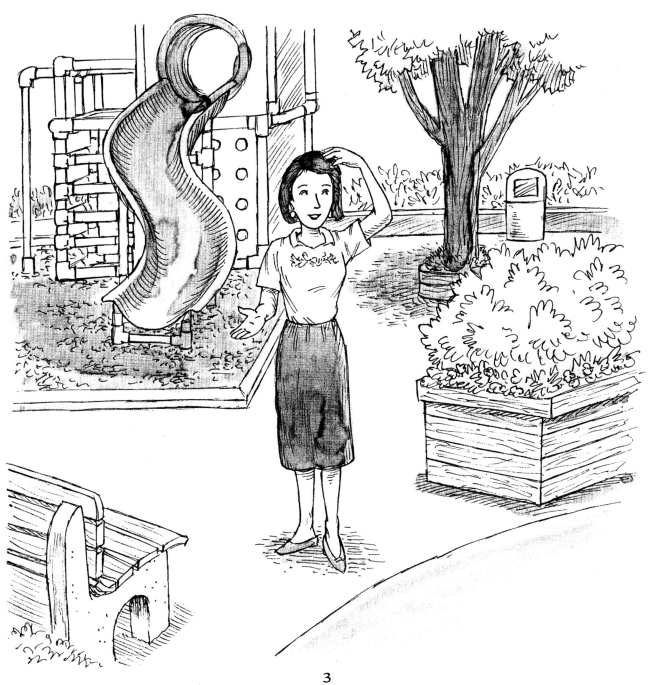

"I'm not in theeeeeere. . .

"I'm not under theeeere. . . "

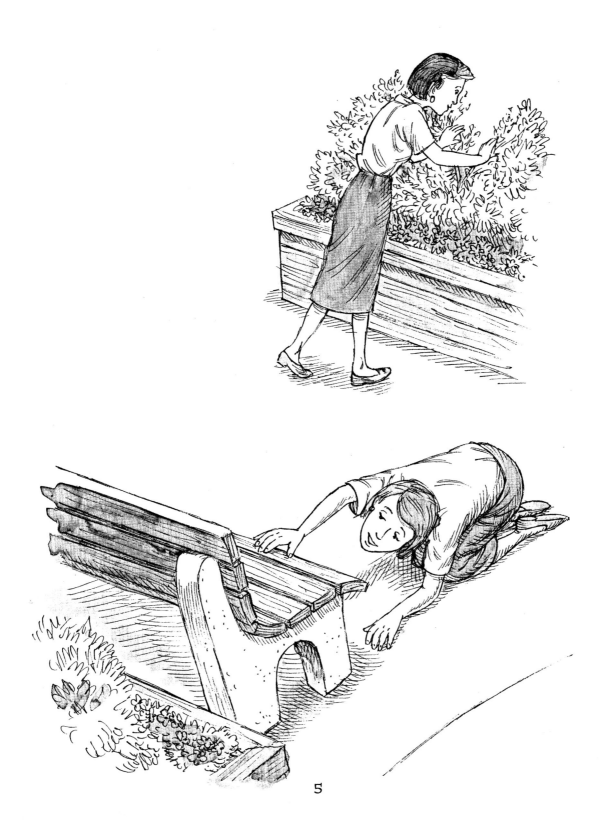

"I hardly ever go behind theeeeere!

"You're never gonna finnnnnnnd mmm— "

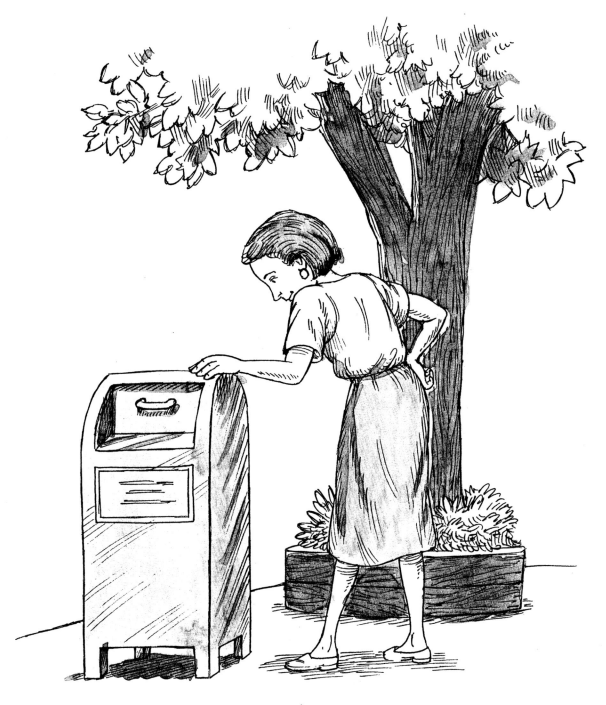

"Oh!" shouts Lilli. "Oh no! You did it! Here I am!! As you can see, I love to hang up-side-down. . . just a minute. . ."

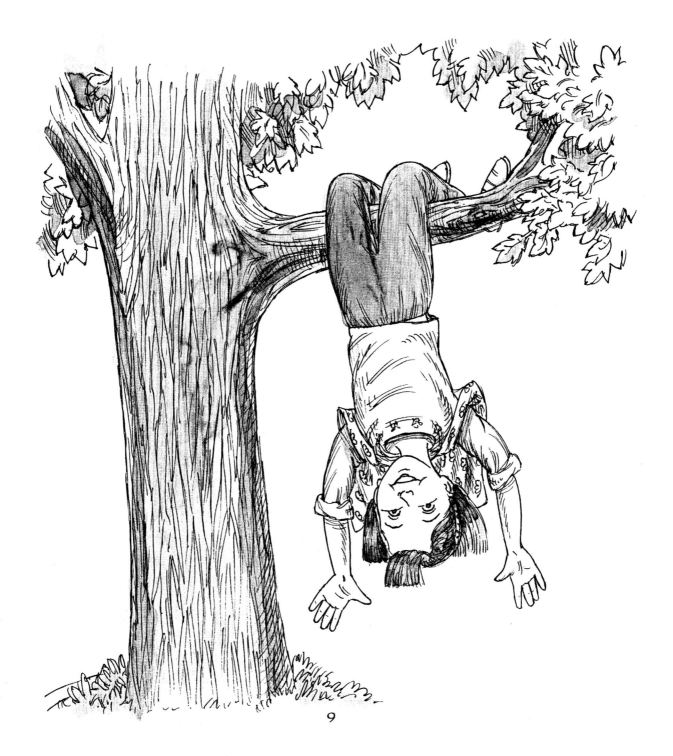

"There! I am a very big girl. I can jump real high, run real fast and sing real loud. You can be my helper(s) today. Now helper(s), let's hear you say, 'LAAAAA!'. . . Louder!. . . Great!

"I have a friend named Walter. He is around here somewhere. Walter is almost as big as me."

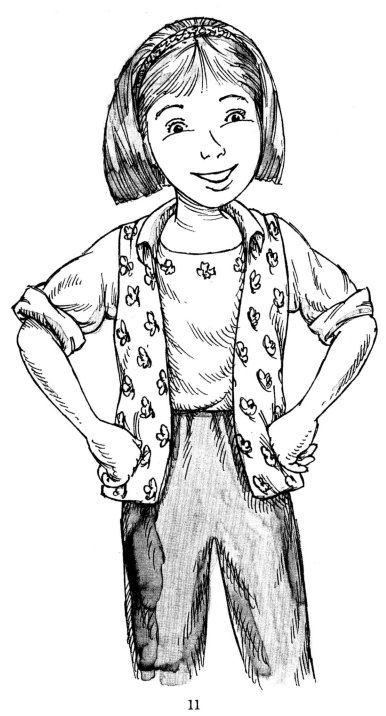

"What!" shouts Walter, jumping out from behind a tree. "I think I am way bigger! Hey helper(s), look at me. . . I can swing and jump from these bars here. . . I can make silly faces too. When I see yucky stuff I make a funny face like this. . .Helper(s), let's see what kind of silly face YOU can make! . . . Good!"

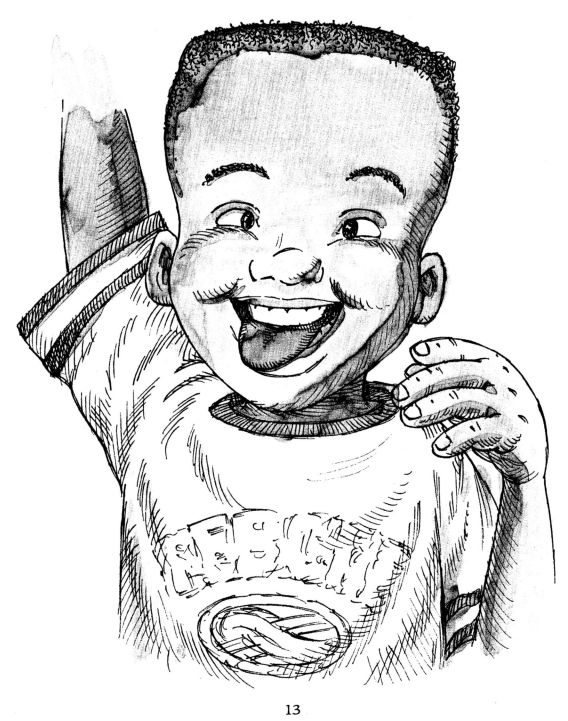

"Hey," says Walter suddenly. "Lilli, didn't you say you were going to tell me about something special today?!"

"That's right!" she answers. "Okay, now first, Walter, tell me what makes you happy."

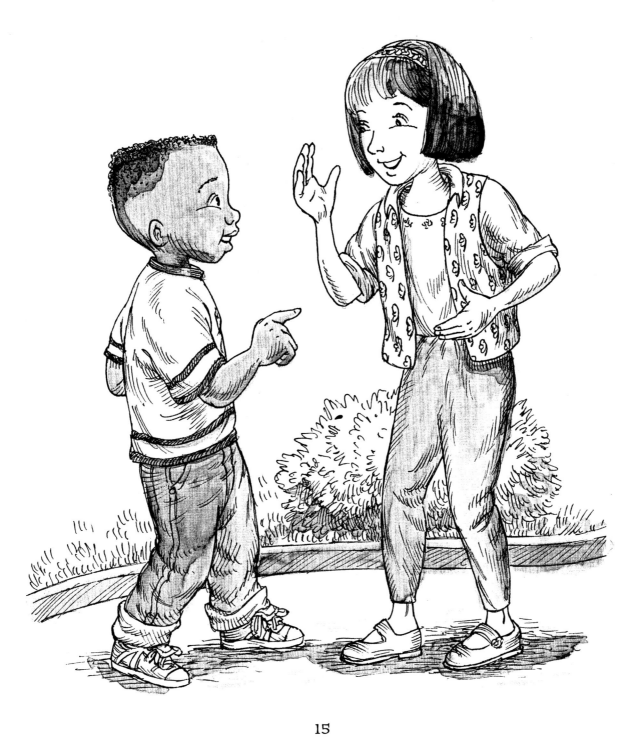

"I know!" answers Walter. "When I go to the park to play with my friends a little part of me feels so happy inside. I say 'WHEEEEEEEEEEEEEE!' when I go down the slide! Helper(s), let's hear you say, 'WHEEEEEEEEEEEEEEEE'. . . Fantastic 'Wheee!'"

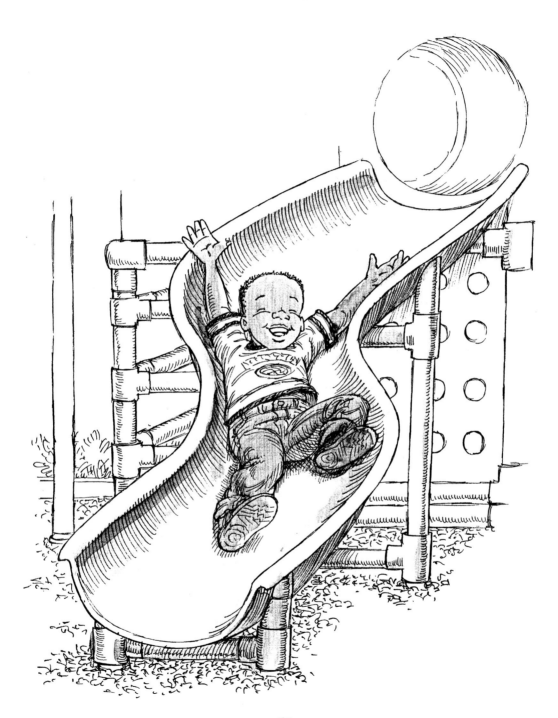

"Walter, can you remember a time you felt scared?" asks Lilli.

"Well," he replies, "on the Fourth of July, when the fireworks go 'BOOM!', a little part of me feels scared inside. But when I get a big hug, that scared part feels much better. Helper(s), make us a big BOOM noise . . . Good!"

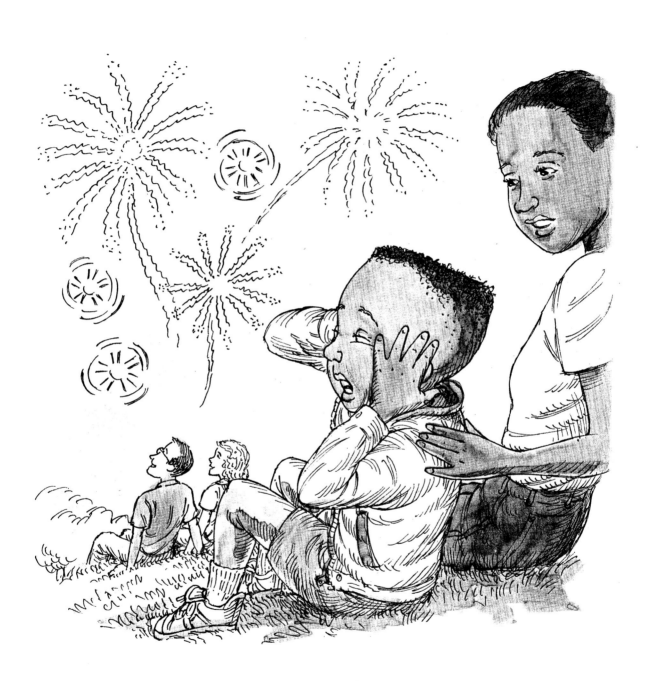

"Being scared or happy are feelings," says Lilli. "Walter, tell me about more kinds of feelings."

"Hmmm. . . ," he thinks. "Oh! I know! Yesterday I asked for ice cream before dinner, but no one would let me have ANY. Boy, a little part of me got SO mad! Even though I know dinner makes me big and strong. Helper(s), show me how big and strong YOU are! Make a muscle and say 'Grrr!' Grrrreat!"

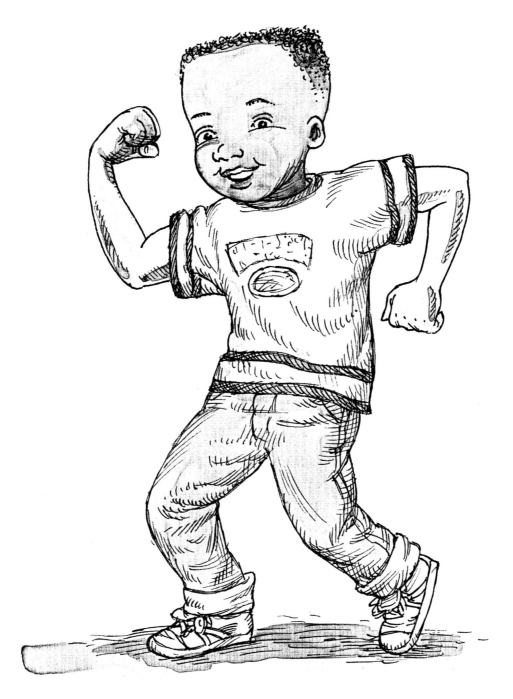

"One time a kid hit me with a toy," remembers Lilli. "Boy, a part of me felt so sad. But when my aunt kissed it better, I stopped crying. Helper(s), say, 'DON'T HIT ME!'. . . Great!"

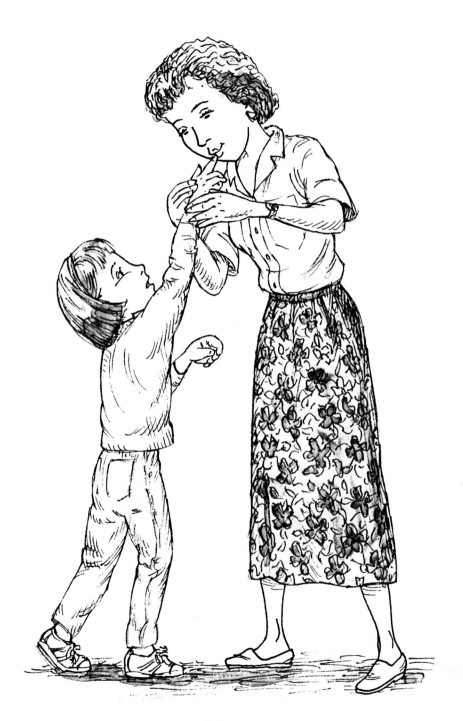

"We have lots of different feelings," says Lilli. "We can even feel different things at the same time. When we have bad or sad feelings it is always good to ask a grownup–someone big–to help us. Helper(s), say, 'HELP ME, I FEEL BAD!'. . .Good!

"Remember to share happy feelings too. Helper(s), say, 'I AM SO HAPPY!'. . . Fantastic!"

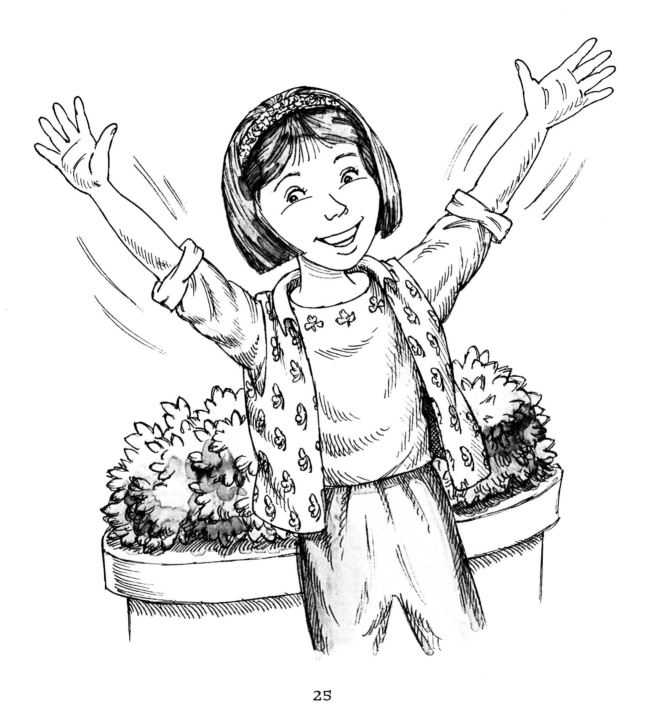

"We love to be hugged by people we love," Lilli says, **"but we don't always like to be touched.** We all have special, private body parts. I am a girl, so my special private body parts are my vagina,* my bottom* and my breasts.*"

*Substitute terms for the formal names of body parts may be used. However, the child should be aware of the appropriate words, even if these are not used regularly.

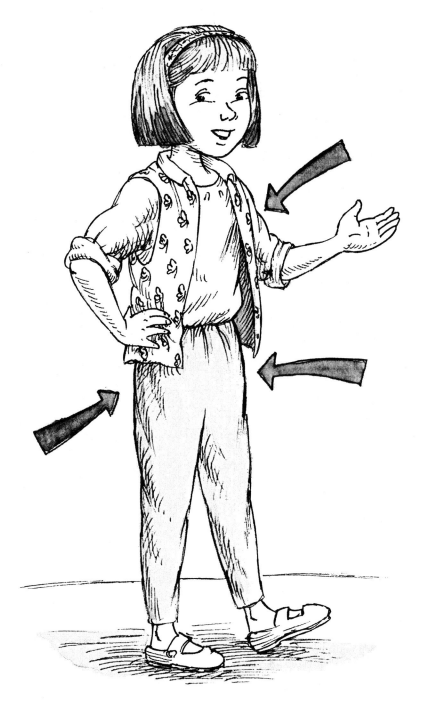

"Well," Walter says, "I am not a girl at all. I am a boy, so my special, private body parts must be my bottom* and my penis.*"

*Substitute terms for the formal names of body parts may be used. However, the child should be aware of the appropriate words, even if these are not used regularly.

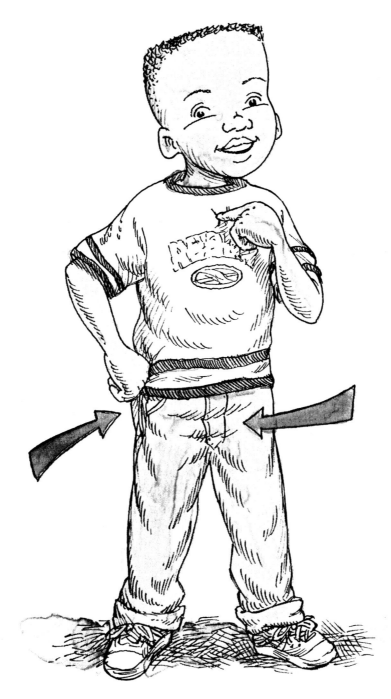

"Right!" says Lilli. "Special body parts are private. They are just for YOU. Your mom or dad or baby sitter can clean your special body parts in the bathtub. Your doctor might check them when she checks the rest of your body. But cleaning and checking are real quick. Except for that, our Body Rules tell us that **little kids never, EVER share their special, private body parts with anyone.**"

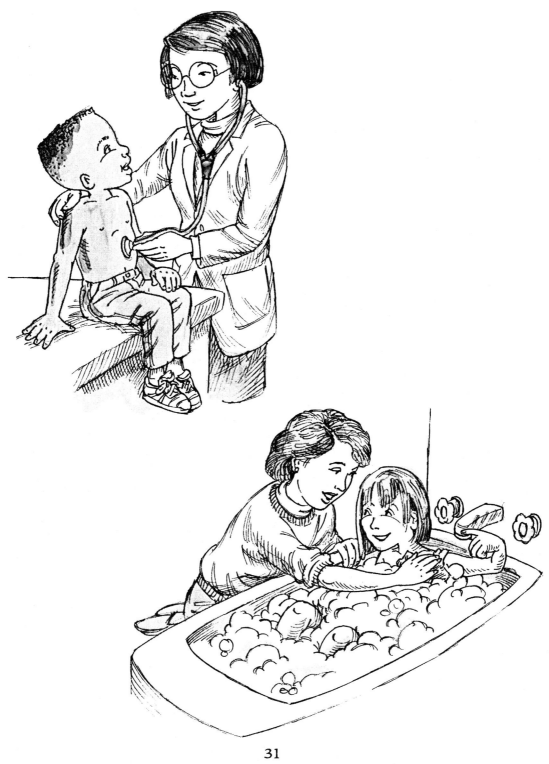

"It makes me think of my special teddy bear Ralph," says Walter. "I sleep with him every night. Mom says I do not have to share Ralph with anyone. He is special and just for me. Private body parts are like that too, **just for me!**"

"Right!" says Lilli. "Kids do not share private body parts. STAND UP, Helper(s), and say a loud, 'NO! DO NOT TOUCH MY PRIVATE PARTS!'. . . Great!"

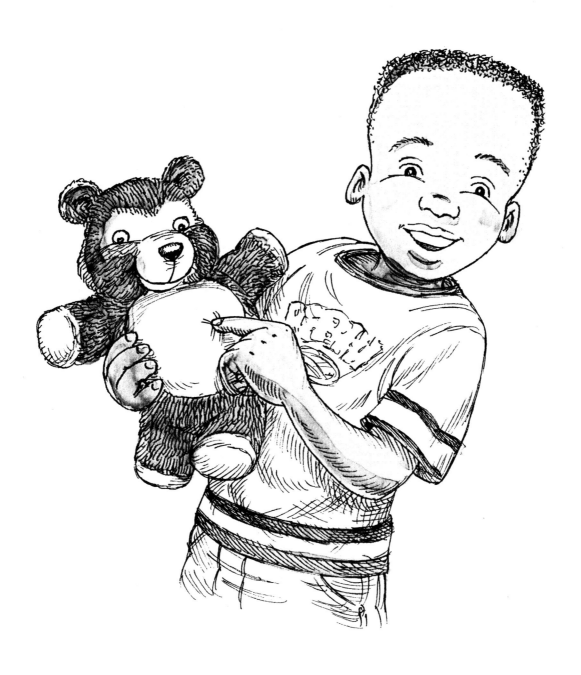

33

"So no one," asks Walter, "not even your mom or dad, aunt or uncle, teacher or baby sitter, neighbor or friend, sister or brother or stranger should touch your private body parts, unless they are supposed to check or clean you quickly?"

"Right!" says Lilli.

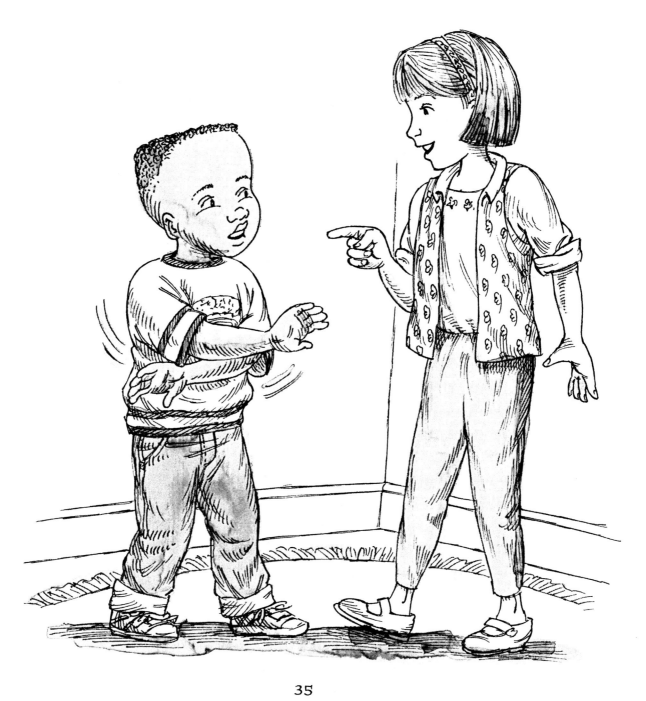

"What if someone wants us to touch **their** private body parts? Should we?" asks Walter.

"NO!"says Lilli, "Little kids DO NOT touch **other people's** special private body parts. We don't touch, rub against or look at anyone's special body parts either–**with anything**, even if a kid or grownup asks or tells us to. Helper(s), stand up again and say a very loud, 'KIDS DO NOT TOUCH OTHER PEOPLE'S PRIVATE BODY PARTS!'. . . Excellent!"

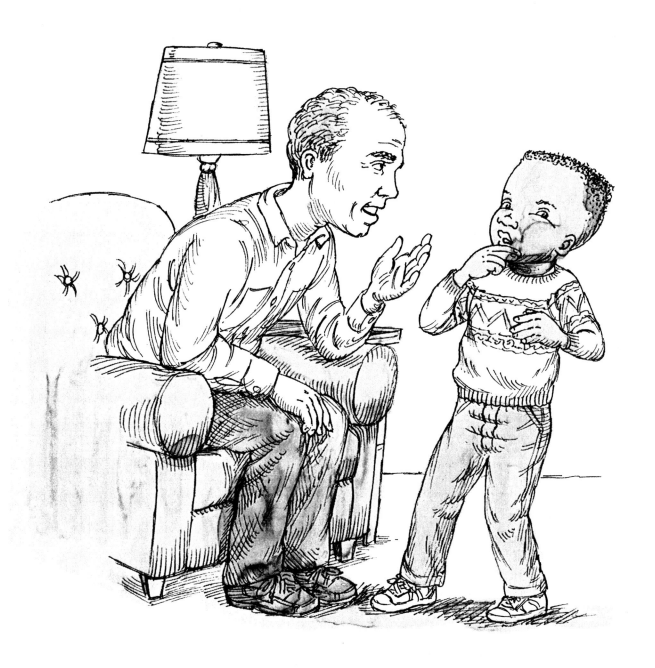

"We also don't let anyone take our picture when we don't have any clothes on," says Lilli, "and we don't look at naked pictures either!"

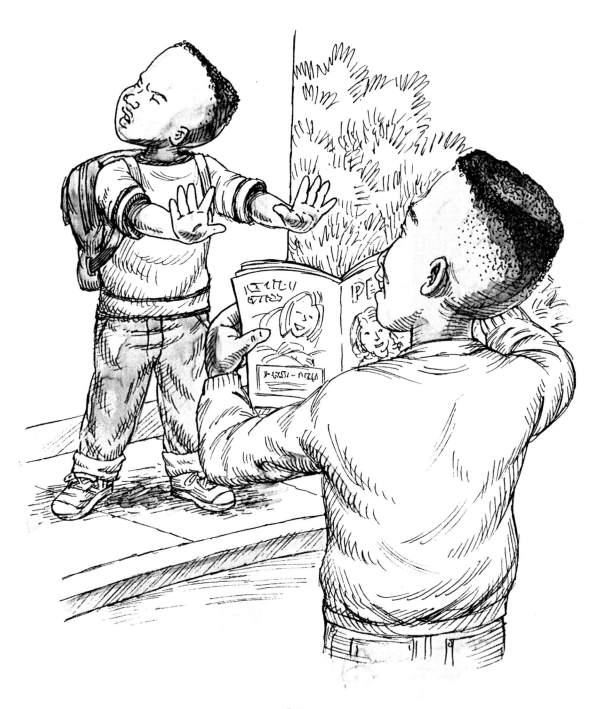

"If someone tries to touch us, should we keep it a secret and not tell anyone?" asks Walter.

"Always tell a grown-up right away, and if you can, go to a safe place." says Lilli. "Tell a teacher or mom or dad or aunt or uncle or policeman or any grown-up. If the grown-up doesn't stop touching you, keep on telling other grown-ups."

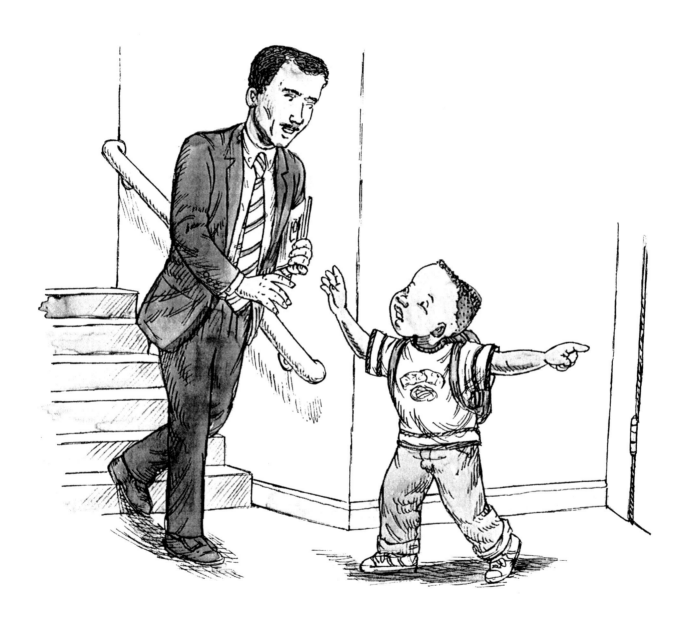

'"What if someone gives me candy or something special so I won't tell or so I'll let them touch me?" asks Walter. "What if they yell or say something mean or scary? That might make a part of me feel bad or scared or sad or shy, and I wouldn't know what to do."

"**Always** stand up and say a loud 'NO!' **Always** tell, no matter what!" answers Lilli. "Helper(s), show me how you can stand up and say a super loud, 'NO!'. . . Great 'NO!'"

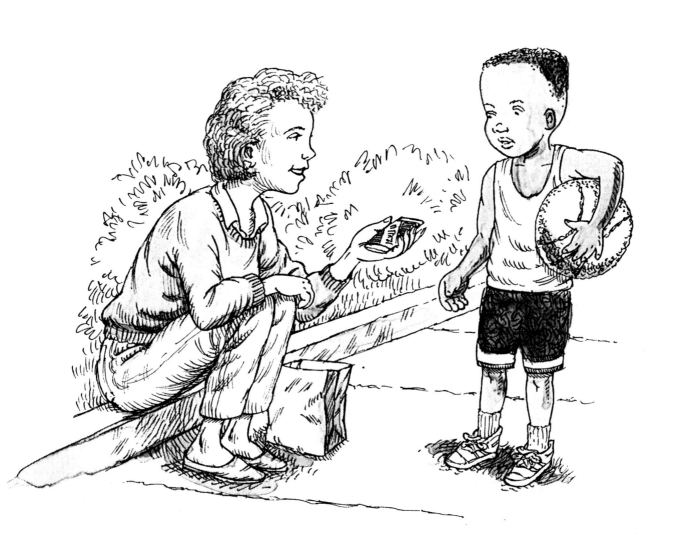

"Hey!"says Walter. "If someone touches or tries to touch our private body parts, and it's **not** to clean or check us quickly, is it OUR fault? What if we liked how it felt? Did we do something wrong?"

"NO!"says Lilli."If a grownup or another kid touches our private body parts, even if they are usually nice, THEY ARE WRONG, AND **WE** ARE NOT! Helper(s), say, 'WE ARE GOOD!'...Great!"

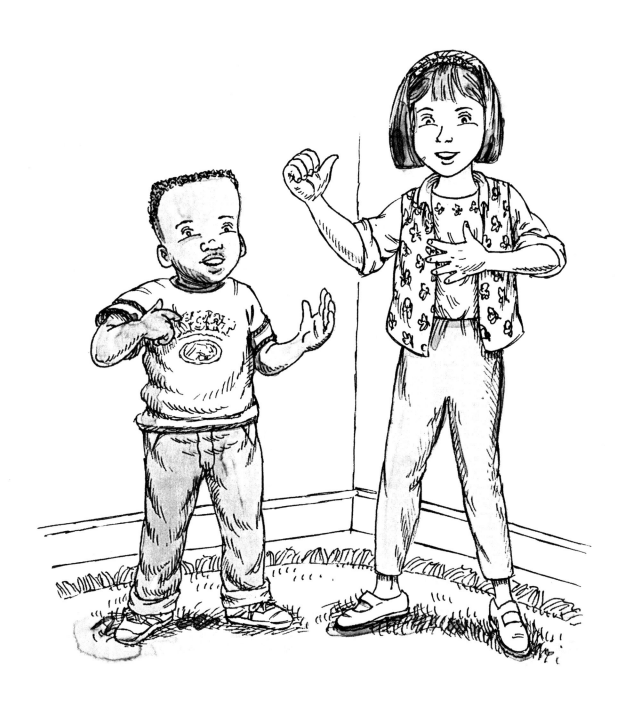

"But," says Walter, "what if someone already touched our private body parts, or asked us to touch them? Or what if we told a grown-up and they did not believe us? What do we do now?"

"ALWAYS TELL A GROWN-UP!" says Lilli, "AND KEEP ON TELLING GROWN-UPS UNTIL THE TOUCHING STOPS FOREVER!

"If a part of you feels bad, scared, sad, or shy, or if you just don't know what to do, **find a grown-up to help you,**" says Lilli.

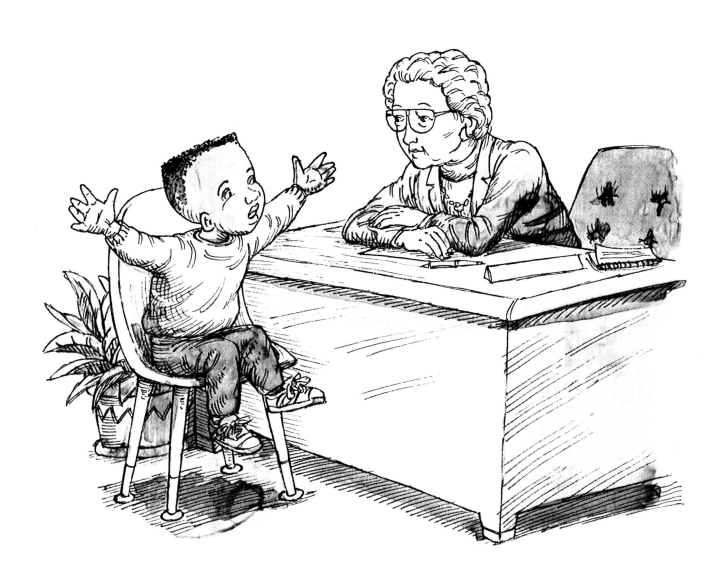

"Grown-ups can help us with bad feelings. Tell your mom or dad or aunts or uncles or teacher or baby-sitter or a policeman, or your friend's mom. Grown-ups can help us with lots of things. That makes us feel so safe and happy! Helper(s), let's hear you say a loud, 'I AM SO HAPPY!' . . . Great!

"I am so happy too!" says Lilli. "Helper(s), you did great! And now we know something really important!

"Thank you for helping me tell Walter about safety! Now you are ready to take our Body Rules Safety Quiz.** You can say goodbye to us for now, but you may want to read our story again soon."

**Due to their limited attention span, younger children should be briefly introduced to an unrelated book or activity before continuing from the story to the quiz. However, it is not mandatory to read both story and quiz on the same day. In fact, the quiz may be omitted altogether if it exceeds the developmental level of the child.

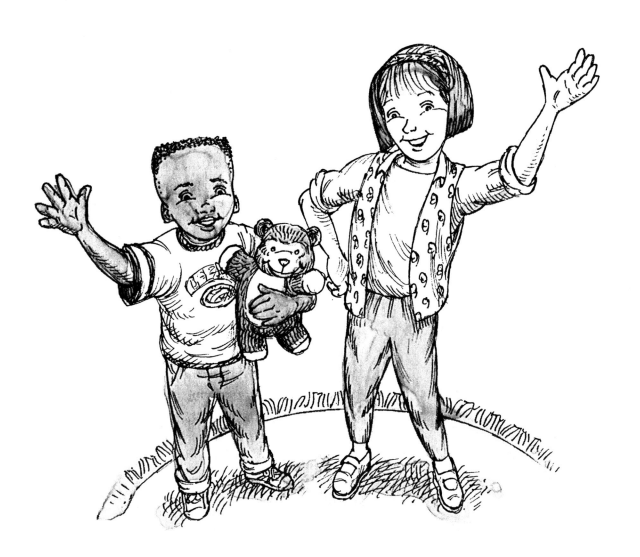

Body Rules SAFETY QUIZ

"Hi there Helper(s)!" says Lilli. "We sure have learned a lot together! Let's see how much we can remember!

"Don't forget, our **special private** body parts are our bottom,* vagina* and breasts* or penis.* **They are just for YOU! No one should touch your special, private parts except if your mom or dad or baby sitter or doctor or someone taking care of you needs to check or clean you quickly. Kids never share** *other people's* **private body parts either, even if a boy or girl or grown-up asks you to.**
Okay, Helper(s), are you ready? . . . Good!

"Is your nose a private body part?"

("NO!")

"Right!" says Lilli. "Are your ears private body parts?"

("NO!")

"Great!" says Lilli. "Is your bottom* a private body part?"

("YES!")

"Fantastic!" says Lilli. "If you are a boy, should someone touch your penis* or your bottom?*"

("NO!")

*Substitute terms for the formal names of body parts may be used. However, the child should be aware of the appropriate words, even if these are not used regularly.

"Good!" says Lilli. "Should you touch someone else's penis* or bottom?*"

("NO!")

"That's right!" says Lilli. "If you are a girl, should someone touch your vagina,* breasts* or bottom?*"

("NO!")

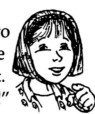

"Excellent!" says Lilli. "Stand up and say: 'NO! DON'T TOUCH MY PRIVATE BODY PARTS!' . . . Fantastic! Say 'I DON'T TOUCH OTHER PEOPLE'S PRIVATE BODY PARTS EITHER!' . . . Great!"

"Remember," reminds Lilli, "if kids or grown-ups try to touch your private body parts, even if they are people you like or love, they are wrong, and **you are right**. Say 'I AM GOOD!'. . . Great!"

"The Kids Body Rules are very important," says Lilli.

1. Kids do not share special private body parts with other kids or grown-ups.

2. Stand up and say a loud 'NO!'

3. If you can, go to a safe place.

4. Tell a grown-up like your mom or dad, grandma or grandpa, neighbor, teacher, or policeman or aunt or uncle right away if someone touches your special body parts.

5. Keep on telling until the touching stops forever.

6. Remember, it is never your fault!

"Now helper(s), if a boy or girl or grown-up tries to touch a kid's private body parts, should you be quiet like this. . .or should you tell a grown-up right away?"

("TELL A GROWN-UP RIGHT AWAY!")

"Right!" says Lilli. "What if the grown-up doesn't believe you or if the touching doesn't stop? Should you be quiet like this. . .or should you keep on telling until the touching stops?"

("KEEP ON TELLING UNTIL THE TOUCHING STOPS!")

"Great!" says Lilli. "If someone scares you or tells you not to tell, or offers you candy or a treat, even if it is a kid or grown-up you like or love, should you take the candy or treat or should you tell a grown-up?"

("TELL A GROWN-UP!")

"Yes, but what if you already took the candy or treat or someone already touched your private parts or already asked you to share their private parts?" asks Lilli. "What should you do?"

("TELL A GROWN-UP!")

"Great!" says Lilli. "What if you are scared or sad or shy or you just don't know what to do? Should you be quiet about the touching like this. . .or should you tell a grown-up?"

("TELL A GROWN-UP!")

"Good!" says Lilli. "Grown-ups can help us with scary or sad feelings! Tell a grown-up and keep telling until the unsafe touching STOPS forever!

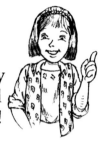

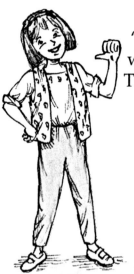

"See how big and strong and smart we are! Now we know how to keep our bodies SAFE! That makes us feel great!"

ADULT GUIDEBOOK FOR PARENTS, CARETAKERS, COUNSELORS, RELATIVES, CLERGY, AND EDUCATORS

Nothing is as important as our children's safety. We constantly give them instructions: "Don't run into the street!"; "Don't talk to strangers!"; "Don't play with fire!" But when it comes to sexual abuse, our children are often unprepared.

Sexual molestation, the abuse of power involving the sexualization of a child, is a problem of growing concern. According to juvenile protection records, in 1993, in the United States alone, approximately 330,000 children were reported victims of sexual abuse (1). In a recent ten-year span, recorded accounts of child molestation increased 2,000 percent (2). Despite these shocking statistics, experts overwhelmingly agree that most child sexual victimization never comes to the attention of the authorities (3–7). Perpetrators are specialists at locating, exploiting and silencing victims. One study found that 403 molesters abused 67,000 youngsters. For every one act in which a perpetrator was caught, 30 acts were committed (3).

Sexual molestation of very young children is more common than once believed. Studies reveal that 25 to 50 percent of all victims may be under the age of seven (28–35). These youngsters are particularly vulnerable because they are trusting, unprepared, and easily manipulated, scared, or shamed into silence. In fact, the sexual assault of a child rarely requires force or violence (4, 12). Because they tend to be undereducated in this area, children, especially young children, are easy targets.

We value respect for authority in our young. In the home, school and community children are taught to obey. They learn to be "good" boys and girls: "Listen to your uncle... Do what the baby sitter tells you." Yet clearly minors need different rules concerning their bodies. Sometimes a youngster must say no, even to an adult or older child. For the abuser, an unaware child is the ideal victim. Community ignorance and fear perpetuate the danger. Someone, besides a potential molester, must begin to talk to small children about their bodies.

Sexual victimization of minors is preventable. Most children and adults can easily be trained to detect and avert such abuse. Research suggests that, when equipped with the proper information, caretakers can be just as, or more effective as teachers and experts in preventing child sexual assault(39).

This book is intended for three- to eight-year-old* children. The goal is to empower and inform both youngsters and adults. The message is simple, straightforward, and in many ways no more complex than the daily safety instructions we routinely teach the young.

*Contingent upon the child's developmental level.

WHAT IS BODY SAFETY?

Personal safety educates children in the following simple, yet essential **Kids Body Rules:**

> 1. Certain parts of our bodies are **special and private.**
> 2. Except for a quick cleaning, we **do not share** our special, private body parts or the special, private body parts of **others.**
> 3. If a kid or grown-up tries to share our or their private body parts **no matter what they say we always:**
>> –**Stand up** and say a loud "NO!"
>> –If you can, go to a safe place.
>> –Tell a grown-up right away, and keep on telling until the unsafe touching stops **forever!**
>> –Remember, it is **never our fault!**

The storybook, *My Body Is Mine, My Feelings Are Mine,* is designed to introduce the essential information that children need for body safety. The Body Rules Safety Quiz at the end of the story is designed to reinforce the learning of these safety behaviors. The book will also help encourage children to talk to appropriate adults whenever they have concerns.

INFORMATION VS. MISINFORMATION

You may be wondering, if prevention is so critical, why isn't it more widely discussed? Although community awareness about child sexual abuse is growing, the prevention movement, in many ways, is still in its infancy. Unfortunately, several misconceptions about child molestation and personal safety still exist. Hopefully, someday soon, more families, schools, counselors, community organizations and health care professionals will work together to end victimization and dispel myths such as those listed below.

SEXUAL ABUSE PREVENTION MYTHS

1) **My child is not exposed to potential abusers.** You might think your child could never be sexually abused. Although we hope this is the case, the information listed below may be of help:

–RICH OR POOR, IT DOESN'T MATTER: Sexual abuse is found at all levels of society and in every ethnic, religious and racial group (3,8–11). Abusers are typically indistinguishable from the general population (3,12). They are everywhere, and they are nowhere. A child molester is just as likely to be well-groomed, sociable and educated as odd or suspicious.

–MOLESTERS ARE LIKELY TO BE SOMEONE YOU KNOW: Only 25 percent of abusers are strangers to their victims (9,11,13,14). In fact, a youngster is more likely to be molested in his or her own home or the home of a relative or acquaintance than in an unfamiliar setting.

–ADULT FEMALE MOLESTERS: Although men are most often thought of as molesters(15–19), research of child sexual abuse in day care settings found females accounted for 40 percent of offenders (20). Female molesters are less likely to admit to abuse (15).

–BOYS ARE AT RISK: Boys (17, 21–24), as well as girls, may be molested. Male victimization is typically under-reported. Although both boys and girls are most likely to be abused in the home, male victims are often molested by someone outside the family (23,56). Girls are more frequently abused by a stepfather (13,57). Abusers of boys tend to be relatively close in age to the victim, and the molestation is often more severe and violent (58–60).

–CHILDREN MOLEST: It is not uncommon for minors, especially victims of sexual abuse, to molest siblings or other youngsters.** Among children of the same age, curiosity about genitalia and limited, unforced touching of each other or themselves is, in most circumstances, normal. However, the child perpetrator molests same age, younger, disabled, older, more naive or less powerful victims. Research suggests that many adult abusers developed perpetrator tendencies during adolescence, often by age fourteen (25) or fifteen (26,27). Teenage offenders tend to commit the most dangerous, extensive type of abuse (61).

–MOLESTERS MAY BE HETEROSEXUAL, HOMOSEXUAL, OR BISEXUAL: Molesters can be of the same or opposite sex as their victim(s). Per perpetrator, men who abuse boys tend to abuse the highest numbers of children (3).

2) **Educating children in personal safety will scare them, or put ideas in their head.**
Does it damage children to teach them not to play with fire or run into the street? These messages all deal with other types of body safety. If we teach children that our bodies

---

**Young victims in particular may try out new, deviant behavior on other children, just as they might share other types of new behavior. This does not necessarily mean the youngster is a "perpetrator."

are not frightening, the notion of privacy will not be frightening either.

3) **Personal safety instruction includes sex education.** Readers of *My Body is Mine, My Feelings Are Mine* may be surprised at the simplicity of the message to children: "You have special, private body parts. Except for a quick cleaning, children do not share their own or touch other's private body parts. Stand up, say a loud NO! and tell a grown-up if someone tries to give you an unsafe touch. If you can, go to a safe place. Keep on telling grown-ups until the touching stops forever. Remember, it is never your fault." Period. It is both inappropriate and unnecessary to teach a young child about sex to educate them in personal safety.

4) **My child is too young to learn about personal safety.** Unfortunately, no child is too young to be sexually abused. Accounts of molestation of infants, toddlers and preschoolers are increasing. Research suggests that up to one-half of child victims are under the age of seven (28– 35), and among the most commonly abused are four-year-olds (2,36–38). Therefore, teaching children to prevent molestation must begin early.

5) **I am not qualified to teach personal safety to a child.** If you care about children, and can calmly talk to a youngster about learning not to share his or her private body parts, then you are qualified. A recent study indicates that parents, not specialists, may be more successful at teaching body safety (39).

6) **Teaching personal safety probably won't do any good anyway.** Perpetrators choose their victims carefully. A child well-trained in body safety, who will say "NO!" and tell an adult, may very well be less likely to be abused. Research suggests that even young children can learn to stop abuse, (40) especially when taught using an interactional approach (41–44) such as offered by Walter and Lilli. In addition, adults educated in prevention can be powerful allies in establishing a safe environment.

RELIEVING OUR ANXIETY

Anxiety is largely a learned response. If we are anxious, our children become uneasy. Our youngsters learn best when we are calm and confident in our approach. The more comfortable we are teaching personal safety, the more comfortable they become protecting themselves. But how do we get there?

It is only natural for parts of us to feel frightened, angry, confused or over-whelmed by the thought of sexual abuse. Discussing body safety can seem embarrassing, or cause discomfort. For some, it may bring back painful memories. *** Yet, for most, teaching personal safety in many ways is like learning to ride a bicycle: It might seem difficult at first, but it quickly becomes second nature.

We must address those parts of our personality that naively believe nothing could ever happen to **our** children. Our "denial part" would have us ignore the potential for abuse. Our "scared part" wants to hide, and our "embarrassed" or "ashamed parts" blindly hope someone else will handle the issue for us. Yet no one is in the unique position you occupy with the children in your care.

Relax these parts of your personality by talking to yourself. Tell yourself that you are capable. Remind yourself of your love for the child. Remember that you can be most helpful if you are strong and open to listening to and teaching the youngster.

HOW TO KEEP CHILDREN SAFE

Although it is impossible to guarantee that a child will be safe from abuse, the following guidelines can be helpful.

Body Safety Tips

1) **Stop body shame; teach body safety.** Do not be ashamed to discuss self protection. Although Walter and Lilli introduce these ideas, it is essential that you, and\or adults close to the child, provide reinforcement through praise and periodic repetition of the basic information. Stress that the youngster should tell you about child unsafe touches, **no matter who was involved or what may have been said.** Perpetrators commonly

---

***For those adults who have been sexually abused as children, discussing personal safety may be difficult, but it can be empowering. Sexual abuse tends to run in families. Many children of adult survivors have been molested (53). If the survivor has not received sufficient therapy, he or she may overreact, or find it difficult to discuss these issues. Further help, including counseling or support, may be necessary. The following organization provides a free referral service, activities, and a newsletter for members, and public speaking and information. Survivors, supporters of survivors and professionals are eligible.

VOICES in Action, Inc. (Victims of Incest Can Emerge Survivors)
P.O. Box 148309
Chicago, IL 60614
(773) 327–1500 or (800) 7–VOICES

Until you are able to discuss prevention with the child, ask another relative, teacher or friend to do so. But if you are an important adult in the youngster's life, or have a lot of contact with children, be sure to get the help you need so that you can become available and vigilant in this process as soon as possible.

turn routine adult\child interaction, such as play, toileting or bathing, into abuse, leaving young children confused or unaware that they have been molested. An offender may use threats or frighten youngsters into secrecy. If the abuser is a parent, close family member or friend, the victim might not think to apply safety rules. Our task is to help children feel proud of their bodies, and be clear about privacy and personal safety.

2) **Be available.** You are probably the most important factor in the prevention of sexual abuse. Your attitude and accessibility regarding personal safety will directly affect the child's learning. If you are **relaxed** and **open**, if you **initiate follow-up discussions** and periodically **remind the child about body safety**, you may decrease the likelihood of abuse, or increase the chance of early disclosure.

3) **Be protective.** A safe child is among caretakers who carefully **monitor their social contacts,** including adult or child family members; neighbors; babysitters; school, church, and community employees; volunteers, friends, and acquaintances; playmates and *their* families, neighbors, friends, and relatives, etc. Gather information about those who have access to the child. Be alert. **Along with the facts, trust your instincts. Ask questions and set rules.** For example, you might decide babysitters cannot entertain their relatives or friends in your home, especially those you do not know or trust. You may instruct babysitters not to take the youngster anywhere, even to their own homes, without your permission, especially if you do not know their family or acquaintances.

    Take a proactive stance. Be assured that the schools and organizations to which you entrust the child conduct routine background and criminal checks on all personnel. Be aware of any criminal sexual behavior of all those who come in contact with the minor. Curtail the youngster's exposure to irresponsible adults and children (i.e. inadequate child supervision, substance abuse, violent behavior, etc.)

    Do not be afraid to advocate for children. Unfortunately, most of us have polite, conflict-avoiding components to our personality, and do not like to make others angry or uncomfortable. Yet nothing is more important than a child's safety. Sometimes it is necessary to offend even those you love or respect to protect a child.

    Take action, and do not stop until you are satisfied a child is not at risk. If you feel uncomfortable about a person or place in the child's life, even if you are not sure why, do not wait until it is too late. Ask questions, and keep on asking. If you remain unsure, consider limiting or suspending the minor's contact with suspect persons or activities until safety can be assured.

4) **Keep talking.** At the conclusion of this book, have a discussion with the child. Ask directly if anyone has touched his or her private body parts, aside from quick, routine cleaning. Be available to discuss reactions or questions regarding body safety. Just as you would any other aspect of his or her safety and well-being, continue to reinforce

these concepts throughout the child's development. Teach the youngster to come to you if he or she feels frightened, confused, guilty, angry or worried, just as she might when he or she is proud or happy. Play "what if" games. Ask, for example, "What would you do if someone tried to touch your private body parts?" Give plenty of positive reinforcement for correct responses. Children learn through repetition and creativity. Converse with, never bore, drill or scare the youngster.

5) **Listen to the child.** Often, abused children later recall having told a caretaker or trusted adult about the offense, sometimes repeatedly, only to be ignored, punished or misunderstood. Such information can be difficult to hear. Alternately, busy adults are not always attuned to a child's every remark. Youngsters may leave hints about their concerns or make disguised disclosures through their behavior. They may become reluctant to be with a trusted friend, relative or babysitter. The child may fear or become angry with someone new in his or her life. "I hate Uncle Leroy" or "Sally is scary. Tell her not to come over again" may or may not be the beginning of some sort of a disclosure. Be attentive to the minor's words and behavior. Calmly and sympathetically offer support and ask questions without jumping to conclusions, becoming overwhelmed or angry (at least in the youngster's presence) or avoiding the topic.

Young children may relate victimization in an unconcerned, offhand manner. The abuse might be a small detail in a story; for example, "My teacher has funny underwear." Children look to grownups to define what is and is not acceptable. When a perpetrator suggests sex is okay, a child may comply without hesitation.

If the victim is somewhat older, or the abuse involved force or violence, the child may be confused or upset. In either case, do not minimize or deny a child's allegations. Irrespective of the minor's attitude, a suspected offense requires further action and should never go ignored.

6) **Ask direct questions. Do not allow yourself to be lulled into a false sense of security because you have read this book with your child(ren) once, twice, or many times.** Nothing can replace periodically asking your child, especially if you become suspicious, the following: "Has anyone touched your private body parts? Has anyone asked you to touch their private body parts?" Even when young children have a basic understanding of privacy and body safety, it is not uncommon for them to simply forget or be too shy or frightened to act or to tell.

HOW TO DETECT A CHILD MOLESTER

It is impossible to screen a potential perpetrator with 100 percent accuracy. A molester may have many, few or none of the characteristics described in this section. Survey those in the child's life and compare them with the following checklist. If one or more item applies to a person with whom the child has had contact, it is possible that abuse has or may occur. However, many of these traits alone may not necessarily be cause for alarm. Some behavior may be truly accidental, or there may be a plausible alternative explanation. More conclusive are disclosures by the child, or the rare witness, medical evidence or perpetrator admission. **It is very rare for a perpetrator to confess and seek help voluntarily, or admit to the behavior once it has been detected.**

Child Abuse Prevention Checklist

1. Does the minor have contact with a person known to have molested children? Perpetrators tend to abuse more than one victim, and misuse each child many times. Although offenders may deny and minimize their behavior, children *are* likely to be at risk in the presence of an untreated molester. For example, if a youngster's maternal grandfather sexually abused the child's mother, grandchildren and other minors may well be at risk. Age, time or a prior prison term typically do not lessen a molester's ability or desire to re-offend.

2. Does the child have contact with an untreated victim of sexual abuse? Victims can become molesters. Especially at risk are untreated adult or child male survivors of sexual molestation.

3. Does the minor have contact with someone you don't trust? Without overreacting, it is important to listen to your instincts about those in the child's life. Too often, after it is too late, a victim's caretaker recalls having had a "funny" feeling about the alleged molester. Remember, an abuser can be someone the child loves or admires, and may appear "normal" in every other respect.

4. Do verbal or nonverbal cues cause you concern about the child's well-being when with a particular adult or minor? Does this person look at the youngster in a suggestive or inappropriate manner that causes you or the child discomfort?

5. Does the minor repeatedly spend unaccounted-for time with someone?

6. Does the minor have contact with someone who appears to be sexually attracted to young children, and\or is interested or involved with child pornography?

7. Does an older child or adult seem unnaturally over-involved with the minor, persistently inviting him or her overnight or to activities that are inappropriate for a youngster? Does this person regularly prolong time with the child, perhaps including activities that have not been pre-approved? Is the child treated as if he or she were an adult?

While it is not uncommon for adults to be very involved with young children, some offenders use minors to replace peer relationships: for example, a relative, baby sitter, or parent who habitually takes a young child to late-night adult movies on a Friday or Saturday night. If the child is an emotional peer, he or she could be, or become, a sexual peer as well.

8. Does the youngster have contact with an adult or child who acts consistently, markedly under-aged? In most instances this is normal adult/child interaction. However, molesters behave younger than their age to become emotional and sexual peers of their victims.

9. Is there an adult who appears to introduce sexuality into his or her relationship with the child? This might entail inappropriate touching or kissing, exhibitionism, voyeurism, or sexualized high contact play or discussion. For example, perpetrators may "wrestle" in an erotic manner with victims, intentionally fondling the child. Some offenders take pictures of minors undressed, or show or "accidentally" leave pornography near the youngster. They may fail to respect the child's privacy, or "inadvertently" show their own body to the child. Such activities are "grooming" devices designed to prepare the child for further victimization.

HOW TO DETECT A VICTIM

It can be as difficult to detect a victim as it is a perpetrator. This is one reason prevention is so critical. A child may have many types of responses to victimization. He or she may act perfectly normal, even in the presence of the offender. It is not uncommon for the victim to love, trust and pursue the molester, even after sex has been introduced. The relationship with the abuser may be so important, and so satisfactory in every other way, that the minor dissociates or refuses to respond to the victimization. It is a self-protective mechanism, effective in temporarily protecting the youngster from the trauma. If the offender is a caretaker, a child may be reluctant to jeopardize this important relationship.

Children often do not reveal abuse at all. Many simply have no one to tell, or have been threatened, coerced or shamed into silence. Others have told, to no avail.

When displaying symptoms of sexual abuse, young children may exhibit one or more of the behaviors listed in this section. However, these only *suggest* victimization. Medical, developmental, interpersonal, psychological or other mutually exclusive explanations must be ruled out. Statements from the child or others may or may not provide additional information, as denial, especially by perpetrators, and often by victims as well, is not uncommon.

Victim Checklist

1. Are there changes in the child's mood, behavior or performance, such as excessive crying or sadness, hyperactivity or behavioral problems?

2. Does the youngster have inexplicable fears or worries, such as nightmares, or other sleep disturbances including insomnia, interrupted slumber or excessive need for sleep? This may include a fear of certain people, known or unknown, or fear of a type of people: i.e., fear of men or children of a particular age.

3. Have you noticed an unusual, unexplained change in the minor's developmental behavior: i.e., sudden under-aged or inappropriately over-aged thoughts or activity?

4. Does the child display sudden, inexplicable, developmentally-inappropriate anger or rage, or an abrupt increase in aggressive or violent behavior?

5. Are there unaccountable changes in the child's appetite? This may include a loss of appetite or compulsive overeating.

6. Have you noticed changes in the child's relationships? He or she may no longer have the same level of interest in friends or relatives, and social ties may deteriorate. The child may even withdraw from primary caretakers, or become overly dependent.

7. Has the youngster begun to keep secrets or have a "secret" friend (63)?

8. Has the child developed an unexplained fear or aversion to a specific person, place or activity (63)?

9. Is the minor neglected, abused, over-controlled or disrespected by his or her family or in the living situation? Does he or she have extended exposure to a chaotic environment (63)?

10. Has the child lost interest in activities that previously brought pleasure?

11. Does it seem the child has lost contact with reality: i.e., his or her imaginary life seriously impairs the youngster's understanding and involvement with reality?

12. Have you noticed a marked or unnatural increase in sexual interest, knowledge or behavior, including sexualized play? Although self-touching and curiosity regarding self and other's genitals is normal, compulsive or ritualistic masturbation or simulated

adult sexuality is not: for example, a young child who positions himself, dolls or others to have intercourse or oral sex.

13. Has the child begun to hate him or herself, to self-mutilate, or to display self-destructive or suicidal thoughts or behavior?

14. Does the child have an increase in physical complaints with no apparent basis, particularly headaches and stomachaches?

15. Have you noticed inexplicable genital trauma, infection, disease or irritation, bloodied or disturbed undergarments, or fears or preoccupation with damage to the child's body?

Do not rule out sexual abuse if a young child says he or she has been abused, but does not display symptoms. Conversely, if one or more of the above symptoms exist without a reasonable alternative explanation and the child claims there has been no abuse, there still may very well be cause for concern.

The above checklist is designed to help you detect some possible signs of the abuse only. Before accusations or a report is made it may be helpful to have the child examined by an impartial and experienced therapist who is prepared to examine not only the child, but the accuser, and the alleged perpetrator.

IF A CHILD HAS BEEN ABUSED

1) **Calm the child.** Be gentle and reassuring. Try to comfort and support the youngster, no matter how sad, confused or angry you or the child feels. Your extreme reactions can overburden the youngster. It is important for adults to be consistently available to the victim. Help the minor feel safe and protected. Explain that he or she is not to blame for the abuse, even if he or she enjoyed parts of it, or learned to request it.****

2) **Listen and ask questions.** Allow the youth to express him or herself. Encourage the child to ask questions and discuss fears, confusion or anger. Calmly ask for additional information. Never end discussion prematurely or interrogate the youngster.

3) **Believe the child.** If a child says that he or she has been abused, unless the circumstances are suspicious, believe it. Most experts agree that it is rare for children to lie

about sexual abuse (46, 51). In the unusual case of a false accusation, typically a troubled adult, not a child, has coached the child toward a false accusation. This most commonly happens in the context of an extremely antagonistic child custody fight (52). Research reveals that the single most important factor in victim recovery is a supportive adult (62).

4) **Ensure safety.** Until you are certain the child is out of danger, suspend the youngster's contact with the alleged molester or molesters and confirm the safety of the other children in your care.

5) **Call the child abuse authorities.** Suspected child sexual abuse, physical abuse and neglect should be reported to the authorities. Anyone can call, including parents and children. Professionals, such as doctors, teachers and counselors, are mandated by law to report suspected abuse. **The phone number for each state is listed in the back of this book.** Even mandated reporters are not responsible for investigating child molestation allegations. These are handled by the authorities. Your only obligation is to report your suspicions and the facts as you know them.

6) **Seek family counseling.** Children and their families should begin counseling as soon as possible. A licensed counselor specializing in the area of child sexual abuse can be useful, especially to help the family through the crisis. Solicit recommendations from respected professionals or acquaintances, or consult the community mental health center in your area. For further information and\or referrals and emergency phone counseling contact ChildHelp USA:

>ChildHelp USA
>15757 N. 78th St.
>Scottsdale, AZ 85260
>1-800-4A CHILD

****Children, especially as they get older, often feel guilt or shame because their bodies have a normal sexual reaction to stimulation. The child may have requested the deviant touching because he or she enjoyed it, found comfort in the closeness, or as an unconscious means of gaining control over an aspect of the victimization. However, children who have not been abused rarely initiate sex. For more specific information on approaching this issue with a minor, see *What Should I Tell the Kids* by Ava L. Siegler (54) and talk to a sexual abuse counselor. In addition, an excellent reference for parents or teachers coping with sexually abused children is *The Sexually Abused Child: A Parent's Guide to Coping and Understanding*, by Kathleen Mach Flynn (63).

7) **Obtain a physical examination.** To rule out injury or disease, the child should be examined by an experienced physician. The youngster's pediatrician, a family physician or a facility specializing in child abuse may be recommended. Although a medical exam is often required by the child abuse authorities, a specific doctor or hospital may be requested.

A trusted, non-abusive parent or relative should be present during the exam to act as the victim's advocate and to provide support and clarification. The relative should discuss the details of the exam beforehand and calmly explain these to the child.

WHAT TO EXPECT AFTER A CHILD ABUSE REPORT

Child sexual abuse is against the law. Protective services and juvenile and criminal court may become involved to ensure the safety of the minor and punish the alleged offender. Depending on the criminal history and severity of the misuse, the perpetrator may be incarcerated or ordered to suspend contact with the victim or relocate. The youngster may be removed from his or her home if the environment is unsafe or the non-offending parent is unfit or unable to protect the child. The victim, molester and family can be mandated to undergo an inpatient or outpatient assessment and\or psychotherapy.

Irrespective of the fate of the offender, children must understand they have done nothing wrong. Explain that the perpetrator, not the youngster, is at fault. Tell the child you are proud of him or her for telling. Discuss his or her feelings and needs. Ask what you can do to help the child feel safe again. Reassure the youngster that you will attempt to keep him or her as protected as possible. If the child's family is supportive, not overwhelmed, in the presence of the youngster, disclosure can be empowering for the victim. The minor's siblings can be a source of support as well if they are comforted by non–offending parents and relatives.

Everyone involved is likely to have extreme reactions. Typically, these only add to the victim's worries. Parents should attempt to calm the parts of their personality that might overreact and become overly angry, sad, confused, rebellious, avoidant or hysterical. They must take care to be stable and available to the child. Although nothing in life can prepare a parent or loved one to deal with the sexual misuse of a child, the adult must take a posture of strength, love and commitment to the victim. Family, marital and individual counseling can be helpful and may be recommended.

Once a call is made to the authorities, if deemed necessary, an investigation will typically begin within 24 hours. Usually a social worker or investigator will meet with the victim, family and suspected perpetrator separately. The worker's job is to ensure the child's safety in cooperation with non-offending family members.

HOW TO READ THE STORYBOOK

How you approach reading this book is important. Treat it as you would any other safety matter you and the child regularly discuss. Be calm, caring, thoughtful and open. Facilitate the conversation. Remember, if the child knows you can be approached on this subject, he or she will feel freer to discuss questions or concerns. If you feel uncomfortable, the youngster will protect you from information you may not want to hear. So relax, and be matter-of-fact.

This picture book is not a bedtime story. It should be read when you have plenty of time. **Read the book yourself first, before you approach the child or children.** After you read the story together, discuss it. Encourage questions. Be certain he or she understands the major points. Help the child take The **Body Rules Safety Quiz** at some point. Let the youngster know you are proud of him or her, and of what he or she has learned. Read the book again another day, always when you and the child or children are relaxed. But most importantly, as you will see, even though this is a sensitive subject, you can still have lots of fun with it too!

REFERENCES

(1) McCurdy, K., and Daro, D. (1993). "Current trends in child abuse reporting and fatalities: The results of the 1993 annual fifty–state survey." Chicago: National Committee for Prevention of Child Abuse. (Available from NCPCA, 332 South Michigan Ave., Suite 1250, Chicago, IL 60604–4357).

(2) American Humane Association. (1988). Highlights of Official Child Neglect and Abuse Reporting 1986. Denver: American Humane Association.

(3) Abel, G.G., Becker, J.V., Mittelman, M., Cunningham-Rathner, J., Rouleau, J. L., and Murphy, W.D. (1987). "Self–reported crimes of non–incarcerated paraphiliacs." Journal of Interpersonal Violence, 2(1), 3–23.

(4) Finkelhor, D. (1984). Child sexual abuse: New theory and research. New York: Free Press.

(5) Finkelhor, D. and Associates (Eds.). (1986). A sourcebook on child sexual abuse. Newbury Park, CA: Sage.

(6) Russell, D.E.H. (1984) Sexual exploitation: Rape, child sexual abuse, and workplace harassment. Beverly Hills: Sage.

(7) Finkelhor, D. (1991). "Child sexual abuse." In M. L. Rosenberg, and M.A. Fenley, (Eds.)Violence in America, (p. 79–94). New York: Oxford University Press.

(8) Russell, D.E.H. (1986). The secret trauma: Incest in the lives of girls and women. New York: Basic Books.

(9) Wyatt G. (1985). "The sexual abuse of Afro–American and White American women in childhood." Child Abuse and Neglect, 9, 507–519.

(10) Finkelhor, D., and Baron L. (1986). "High risk children." In D. Finkelhor and Associates (Eds.). Sourcebook on child sexual abuse. Newbury Park CA: Sage.

(11) Finkelhor, D., Hotaling, G., Lewis, I.A., and Smith, C. (1990). "Sexual abuse in a national survey of adult men and women: prevalence, characteristics, and risk factors." Child Abuse and Neglect, 14, 19–28.

(12) Crewdson, J. (1988). By silence betrayed: Sexual abuse of children in America. Boston: Little, Brown.

(13) Russell, D. E. H. (1983). "The incidence and prevalence of intrafamilial and extrafamilial sexual abuse of female children." Child Abuse and Neglect, 7, 133–146.

(14) Siegel, J. M., Sorenson, S. B., Golding, J. M., Burnam, M. A., and Stein, J. A. (1987). "The prevalence of childhood sexual assault: The Los Angeles epidemiologic catchment area project." American Journal of Epidemiology, 126, 1141–1153.

(15) Allen, C.M. (1990). "A comparative analysis of women who sexually abuse. Final report." National Center of Child Abuse and Neglect, Washington, D.C.

(16) Elliott, M. (Ed.). (1994). Female sexual abuse of children. NY: Guilford Publications.

(17) Mathews, R. Matthews, J. and Speltz, K. (1991). "Female sexual offenders: A typology." In Patton, M.Q. (Ed.). Family Sexual Abuse: Frontline research and evaluation (pp. 199– 219). Newbury Park: Sage Publications.

(18) Rowan, E.L., Rowan, J.B., and Langelier, P. (1990). "Women who molest." Bulletin of the American Academy of Psychiatry and the Law, 18(1), 79–83.

(19) Wakefield, H., and Underwager, R.C. (1991). "Female child sexual abusers: A critical review of the literature." American Journal of Forensic Psychology, 9(4), 43–69.

(20) Finkelhor, D., and Meyer Williams, L., with Burns, N. (1988). Nursery crimes: Sexual abuse in day care. Newbury Park: Sage Publications.

(21) Finkelhor, D., and Russell, D. (1984). "Women as perpetrators: Review of the evidence." In D. Finkelhor, (Ed.). Child sexual abuse: New theory and research (pp. 171–187). NewYork: Plenum Press.

(22) Faller, K.C. (1987). "Women who sexually abuse children." Violence and Victims, 2(4), 263–276.

(23) Faller, K.C. (1989). "Characteristics of a clinical sample of sexually abused children: How boy and girl victims differ." Child Abuse and Neglect, 13, 281–291.

(24) McCarty, L.M. (1986). Mother–child incest: Characteristics of the offender. Child Welfare, 65, 447–458.

(25) Becker, J. V., Kaplan, M. S., Cunningham–Rathner, J., and Karoussi, R. (1986). "Characteristics of adolescent sexual perpetrators: Preliminary findings." Journal of Family Violence, I, 85–97.

(26) Abel, G. G., Mittelman, M. S., and Becker, J. V. (1985). "Sexual offenders: Results of assessment and recommendations for treatment." In H. H. Ben–Aron, S. I. Hucker, and C. D. Webster (Eds.), Clinical criminology: Current concepts (pp. 191–205). Toronto: M & M Graphics.

(27) Becker, J. V., Cunningham–Rathner, J., and Kaplan, M. S. (1986). "Adolescent sexual offenders: Demographics, criminal and sexual histories, and recommendations for reducing future offenses." Journal of Interpersonal Violence, I, 431–445.

(28) Berliner, L. and Stevens, D. (1982). "Clinical issues in child sexual abuse." Journal of SocialWork and Human Sexuality, I, 93–108.

(29) Cupoli, J. M., and Sewell, P. M. (1988). "One thousand fifty–nine children with a chief complaint of sexual abuse." Child Abuse and Neglect, 12, 151–162.

(30) Faller, K. C. (1988). Child sexual abuse: An inter–disciplinary manual for diagnosis, case management, and treatment. New York: Columbia University Press.

(31) Jaudes, P. K. and Morris, M. (1990). "Child sexual abuse: Who goes home?" Child Abuse and Neglect, 14, 61–68.

(32) Jenny, C., Sutherland, S. E., and Sandahl, B. B. (1986). "Developmental approach to preventing the sexual abuse of children." Pediatrics, 78, 1034–1038.

(33) Lang, R. A., Rouget, A. C., and van Santen, V. (1988). "The role of victim age and sexual maturity in child sexual abuse." Annals of Sex Research, I, 467–484.

(34) Mannarino, A. P., and Cohen, J. A. (1986). "A clinical–demographic study of sexually abused children." Child Abuse and Neglect, 10, 17–23.

(35) Mian, M., Wehrspann, W., Klajner–Diamond, H., LeBaron, D., and Winder, C. (1986). "Review of 125 children six years of age and under who were sexually abused." Child Abuse and Neglect, 10, 223–229.

(36) DeJong, A. R., Hervada, A. R., and Emmett, G. A. (1983). "Epidemiologic variations in childhood sexual abuse." Child Abuse and Neglect, 7, 155–162.

(37) Eckenrode, J., Munsch, J., Powers, J., and Doris, J. (1988). "The nature and substantiation of official sexual abuse reports." Child Abuse and Neglect, 12, 311–319.

(38) Tilelli, J. A., Turek, D., and Jaffe, A. C. (1980). "Sexual abuse of children: Clinical findings and implications for management." New England Journal of Medicine, 320, 319–323.

(39) Finkelhor, D., Asdigian, N., Dziuba–Leatherman, J. (1993). "Victimization prevention training in action: A national survey of children's experiences coping with actual threats and assaults." Family Research Laboratory, University of New Hampshire.

(40) Hill, J.L., and Jason, L.A. (1987). "An evaluation of a school–based child sexual abuse primary prevention program." Psychotherapy Bulletin, 22, 36–38.

(41) Stilwell, S.L., Lutzker, J.R., and Green, B.F. (1988). "Evaluation of a sexual abuse prevention program for preschoolers." Journal of Family Violence, 3, 269–281.

(42) Harvey, P., Forehand, R., Brown, C., and Holmes, T. (1988). "The prevention of sexual abuse: Examination of the effectiveness of a program with kindergarten–age children." Behavior Therapy, 19, 429–435.

(43) Ratto, R., and Bogat, G.A. (1990). "An evaluation of a preschool curriculum to educate children in the prevention of sexual abuse." Journal of Community Psychology, 18, 289– 297.

(44) Wurtele, S.K. (1990). "Teaching personal safety skills to four–year–old children: A behavioral approach." Behavior Therapy, 21, 25–32.

(45) Burgess, A.W., Groth, A.N., Holmstrom, L.L., Sgroi, S.M. (1978). The sexual assault of children and adolescents. Lexington, MA: Lexington Books.

(46) Faller, K. C. (1984). "Is the child victim of sexual abuse telling the truth?" Child Abuse and Neglect, 8(4), 473–481.

(47) MacFarlane, K., and Waterman, J. (1986). Sexual abuse of young children. New York: Guilford Press.

(48) Rieser, M. (1991). "Recantation in child sexual abuse cases." Child Welfare, 70(6), 611–621.

(49) Salter, A. C. (1988). "Epidemiology of child sexual abuse," In W. O'Donohue and J. Geer, The sexual abuse of children: Theory and research, Volume 1, (pp. 1108–138). Hillside, New Jersey: Lawrence Erlbaum Associates, Inc.

(50) Sgroi, S. (1982). Handbook of clinical intervention in child sexual abuse. Lexington, MA: Lexington Books.

(51) Walker, L.E.A. (1988). Handbook on sexual abuse of children: Assessment and treatment issues. New York: Springer.

(52) Jones, D. and McGraw, J.M. (1987). "Reliable and fictitious accounts of sexual abuse in children." Journal of Interpersonal Violence, March, 2(1), pp. 27–45.

(53) Faller, K.C. (1989). "Why sexual abuse? An exploration of the intergenerational hypothesis."Child Abuse and Neglect, 13(4), 543–548.

(54) Seigler, Ava, L. (1993). What should I tell the kids?. New York: Dutton (pp. 238–247).

(55) Wyatt, G.E. and Powell, G.J. (1988). "Identifying the lasting effects of child sexual abuse: An overview." In G.E. Wyatt and G.J. Powell, Lasting Effects of Child Sexual Abuse (pp. 11–17). Newbury Park: Sage.

(56) Kercher, G. and McShane, M. (1984). "Characterizing child sexual abuse on the basis of a multi–agency sample." Victimology, 9(3–4), 364–382.

(57) Kendall, K.A. and Simon, A.F. (1992). "A comparison of the abuse experiences of male and female adults molested as children." Journal of Family Violence, 73(1), 57–62.

(58) Gordon, M. (1990). "Males and females as victims of childhood sexual abuse: An examination of the gender effect." Journal of Family Violence, 5(4), 321–331.

(59) Dube, R. and Hevert, M. (1988). "Sexual abuse of children under 12 years of age: A review of 511 cases." Child Abuse and Neglect, 12(3), 321–330.

(60) Rosenthal, J.A. (1988). "Patterns of reported child abuse and neglect." Child Abuse and Neglect, 12(12), 263–271.

(61) Margolin, L. and Craft, J.L. (1990). "Child abuse by adolescent caregivers." Child Abuse and Neglect, 14(3), 365–373.

(62) Gilgun, J.F. (1990). "Factors mediating the effects of childhood maltreatment." In M. Hunter (Ed.), The sexually abused male; Prevalence, impact and treatment, Vol. 1 (pp. 177–190). Lexington, MA: Lexington Books.

(63) Mach Flynn, K. (1994). The Sexually Abused Child: A Parent's Guide to Coping and Understanding. Williamsburg: Family Insight Books.

CHILD ABUSE REPORTING AGENCIES

ALABAMA
Division of Family Services
50 North Ripley Street
Montgomery, AL 36130
(334) 242-9500

ALASKA
Department of Health and Social Services
Division of Family and Youth Services
PO Box 110630
Juneau, AK 99811
(800) 478-4444
(907) 465-3170

ARIZONA
Department of Health and Social Services
Administration for Children, Youth, and Families
PO Box 44240
Phoenix, AZ 85064
(888) SOS-CHILD

ARKANSAS
Arkansas State Police
Child Abuse Services
1 State Police Plaza Drive
Little Rock, AR 72209
(800) 482-5964 (24 hours)

CALIFORNIA
Department of Social Services
Office of Child Abuse Prevention
744 P Street
M.S. 19-82
Sacramento, CA 95814
(916) 445-2832

COLORADO
Department of Social Services
Division of Children, Youth, and Family
1700 Lincoln Avenue
Denver, CO 80236

(303) 727-3666
(303) 983-6111 (24 hours)

CONNECTICUT
Department of Human Resources
Department of Children and Families
Intake Services
PO Box 882
Middletown, CT 06457
(800) 842-2288 (24 hours)

DELAWARE
Department of Health and Social Services
Division of Youth and Protective Services
321 East 11th Street
Wilmington, DE 19801
(800) 292-9582 (24 hours)
(302) 577-6550

DISTRICT OF COLUMBIA
D.C. Police Department
Youth Division
1700 Rhode Island Avenue N.E.
Washington, D.C. 20018
(202) 671-7233

FLORIDA
Florida Protective Service System
Abuse Registry
2729 Fort Knox Blvd.
Executive Center
Tallahassee, FL 32308
(800) 96-ABUSE (24 hours)
(904) 487-2625

GEORGIA
Department of Human Resources
Division of Family and Children Services
Georgia Protective Office
2 Peachtree Street, Suite 18-470
Atlanta, GA 30303
(404) 657-3408

HAWAII
Department of Social Services
Family and Children Services
Protective Services Intake
420 Waiakamilo Road, Suite 300A
Honolulu, HI 96814
(800) 832-5300 (24 hours)
(808) 587-3300

IDAHO
Department of Health and Welfare
Interstate Compact
PO Box 83720
Boise, ID 83720-0036
(208) 334-5692 (reports are made directly to regional offices)

ILLINOIS
Department of Children and Family Services
Division of Child Protection
State Central Register
406 E. Monroe
Springfield, IL 62701
(800) 25-ABUSE (24 hours)
(217) 785-4010

INDIANA
Division of Family and Children
Social Services
402 W. Washington, Room W364
Indianapolis, IN 46204
(800) 562-2407 (24 hours)
(317) 232-4430

IOWA
Department of Human Services
Child Protective Services
Hoover State Office Building
Des Moines, IA 50319
(800) 362-2178 (24 hours in-state)
(515) 281-3240 (24 hours out-of-state)

KANSAS
Department of Social and Rehabilitation Services
Child Protective and Family Services
Docking Building
915 S.W. Harrison Street
Topeka, KS 66612
(800) 922-5330
(785) 296-0044

KENTUCKY
Cabinet for Families and Children
Department for Community-Based Services
275 East Main Street
Frankfort, KY 40621
(800) 752-6200 (24 hours)
(502) 564-2136

LOUISIANA
Department of Social Services
Division of Community Services
1913 North Street
PO Box 1588
Baton Rouge, LA 70802
(225) 925-4571

MAINE
Department of Human Services
Children's Emergency Services
221 State Street Station 11
Augusta, ME 04333
(800) 452-1999 (24 hours)
(207) 289-2983 (24 hours)

MARYLAND
Department of Human Resources
Child Abuse Screening Unit
Protective Services
312 East Oliver Street
Baltimore, MD 21202
(800) 332-6347

MASSACHUSETTS
Executive Office of Human Services
Department of Social Services
24 Farnsworth Street
Boston, MA 02114
(800) 792-5200 (24 hours)
(617) 748-2000
(617) 232-4882

MICHIGAN
Family Independence Agency
235 South Grand Avenue
Suite 510
Lansing, MI 48909
(800) 942-4357
(517) 373-3572

MINNESOTA
Department of Human Services
Family and Children's Services
444 Lafayette Road
St. Paul, MN 55155-3830
(612) 296-2217

MISSISSIPPI
Department of Public Welfare
Division of Social Services
750 N. State Street
PO Box 352
Jackson, MS 39205
(800) 222-8000
(601) 359-4991

MONTANA
Department of Public Health and Human Services
Child and Family Services Division
PO Box 8005
Helena, MT 59604-8005
(800) 332-6100
(406) 444-5900 (reports are made directly to districts)

NEBRASKA
State Department of Health and Human Services
State Office Building
301 Centennial Mall South
PO Box 95044
Lincoln, NE 68509-5026
(800) 652-1999
(402) 471-3121

NEVADA
Department of Human Resources
Child Protective Services
711 East 5th Street
Carson City, NV 89710
(800) 992-5757 (24 hours)
(775) 864-4422 (reports are made directly to districts)

NEW HAMPSHIRE
Department of Health and Human Services
Division for Children, Youth, and Families
Health and Welfare Building
6 Hazen Drive
Concord, NH 03301
(800) 894-5533 (24 hours)
(603) 271-4714

NEW JERSEY
Department of Human Services
Division of Youth and Family Services
Office of Child Abuse Control
CN 717
Trenton, NJ 08625-0717
(800) 792-8610 (24 hours)

NEW MEXICO
Child, Youth, and Families Department
Social Service Division
Children's Bureau
Pera Building, Room 224
PO Drawer 5160
Santa Fe, NM 87502
(800) 432-2075
(505) 841-6100

NEW YORK
Department of Social Services
N.Y. Child Protective Services
40 N. Pearl Street
Albany, NY 12243
(800) 342-3720 (24 hours)
(518) 474-8740

NORTH CAROLINA
Department of Human Resources
Division of Social Services
Child Protective Service Unit
325 N. Salisbury Street
Raleigh, NC 27603
(919) 733-4622

NORTH DAKOTA
Department of Human Services
Social Services
Child and Family Services
600 East Blvd. Avenue
State Capitol Building
Bismarck, ND 58505
(800) 245-3736
(701) 224-2316 (reports are made directly to regional offices)

OHIO
Department of Human Services
Child Protective Services Unit
Bureau of Child and Adult Protection
65 E. State, Fifth Floor
Columbus, OH 43215
(614) 466-9824

OKLAHOMA
Department of Human Services
Division of Child Welfare
PO Box 25352
Oklahoma City, OK 73125
(800) 522-3511 (24 hours)
(405) 767-2800

OREGON
Department of Human Resources
Children's Services Division
500 Summer Street N.E.
Salem, OR 97310-1017
(800) 854-3508
(503) 378-6704

PENNSYLVANIA
Department of Public Welfare
Child Line
Hillcrest Building 53
PO Box 2675
Harrisburg, PA 17105-2675
(800) 932-0313 (24 hours)
(717) 783-8744

PUERTO RICO
Department of Social Services
Family Services
PO Box 11398, Fernandez Juncos Station
Santurce, PR 00910
(800) 981-8333
(787) 749-1333

RHODE ISLAND
Department for Children and Their Families
Building 7
610 Mt. Pleasant Avenue
Providence, RI 02908
(800) RI-CHILD (24 hours in-state)
(401) 457-4996

SOUTH CAROLINA
Department of Social Services
State Child Protective and Preventive Services Unit
PO Box 1520
Columbia, SC 29202-9988
(803) 898-7318

SOUTH DAKOTA
Department of Social Services
Capitol Building
700 Governors Drive
Pierre, SD 57501-2291
(605) 773-3227

TENNESSEE
Department of Human Services
Protective Services
1000 2nd Avenue North
PO Box 1135
Nashville, TN 37202-1135
(615) 329-1911 (24 hours)
(615) 253-1400 (or local county office)

TEXAS
Department of Human Services
Protective Services for Children Branch
Child Abuse Hotline
PO Box 149030 (MCE-206)
Austin, TX 78714-9030
(800) 252-5400 (24 hours in-state)
(512) 834-3784

UTAH
Division of Child and Family Services
Child Abuse and Neglect Prevention
120 N 200 W, PO Box 45500
Salt Lake City, UT 84145
(800) 678-9399
(801) 538-4100

VERMONT
Agency of Human Services
Division of Social Services
103 N. Main Street
Waterbury, VT 05671-2401
(800) 649-5285
(802) 241-2100

VIRGINIA
Department of Social Services
Bureau of Child Protective Services
730 E. Broad Street
Richmond, VA 23219
(800) 552-7096 (24 hours)
(804) 786-8536

WASHINGTON
Social and Health Services
Bureau of Children's Services
PO Box 45710
Olympia, WA 98504
(800) 562-5624

WEST VIRGINIA
CRISS-CROSS, Inc.
115 South 4th Street
Clarksburg, WV 26301
(800) 352-6513
(800) 422-4453

WISCONSIN
Department of Health and Family Services
PO Box 7851
Madison, WI 53707
(608) 266-3036 (reports are made directly to local county offices)

WYOMING
Department of Family Services
Hathaway Building, 3rd Floor
Cheyenne, WY 82002-0490
(800) 457-3659
(307) 777-7564 (reports are made directly to local county offices)

ABOUT THE AUTHOR

Susan L. Hoke is a licensed clinical social worker, activist, workshop leader and therapist specializing in the prevention of family violence and child sexual abuse. She is an adjunct faculty member at the Institute of Juvenile Research at the University of Illinois School of Medicine. She was recently selected as Chicago Social Worker of the Year by the National Association of Social Workers. She is the mother of an active five-year-old, the inspiration for her current book.

ORDER THESE AND MANY OTHER THERAPEUTIC STORY BOOKS
FROM CHILDSWORK/CHILDSPLAY, LLC

Sometimes I Drive My Mom Crazy, But I Know She's Crazy About Me
This warm, humorous, and true-to-life story of a young AD/HD boy addresses the many difficult and frustrating issues that kids like him confront every day—from sitting still in the classroom, to remaining calm, to feeling "different" from other children. This book takes an amusing look at how this youngster develops a sense of self-worth by learning to deal with his problems with the help of the adults who care about him. Hailed by parents and educators as one of the best books written to help motivate AD/HD children to cope with their problem in a positive way. Paperback. Ages 6-12.

The Very Angry Day That Amy Didn't Have
Margaret and Amy are two girls in the same class who coincidentally are both having a very difficult day. But Margaret always makes things worse by her negative reactions, making people mad at her, while Amy finds positive ways to solve the various problems she encounters. This simple but poignant book is an excellent tool to help young children learn alternatives to getting angry. Paperback. For ages 4-10.

Jumpin' Jake Settles Down: A Workbook to Help Impulsive Children Learn to Think Before They Act
This hilariously-illustrated story and activity book tells how Jake changes from an itchin-kind-of-frog to a responsible thinkin'-kind-of-frog. The book features 50 activities that help children learn cognitive techniques and behavioral skills to control their impulsivity. Paperback. For ages 5-10.

Face Your Feelings!
This book includes 52 pictures of children, teens, adults, and older adults, expressing the feelings that children are most concerned about. With each picture, the person tells about the kinds of things that made him/her feel that way. Includes a mylar mirror to help children "face their own feelings." Paperback. Ages 3 and up.

The Building Blocks of Self-Esteem
Self-esteem is more than just self-love. It's a deep sense of self-worth based on the mastery of specific traits and skills which help children succeed and develop positive relationships with others. This workbook is filled with activities that form a multi-modal approach to improving a child's self-esteem: Affect, Behavior, Cognition, Developmental, Education, Social System. Paperback. Ages 5-12.

TO ORDER, OR FOR A FREE CATALOG OF BOOKS AND GAMES THAT ADDRESS THE MENTAL HEALTH PROBLEMS OF CHILDREN, CALL:

Childswork/Childsplay, LLC
1-800-962-1141